Journey into a ...

Disturbed Mind

Grateful
Steps

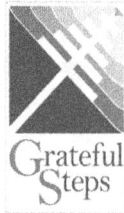

Grateful Steps Foundation
159 South Lexington Avenue
Asheville, North Carolina 28801

Copyright © 2014 by Earl Lynn Surrett
Library of Congress Control Number 2014939529
Surrett, Earl Lynn
Journey into a Disturbed Mind

Design of cover graphic of author by Michele Scheve
ISBN 978-1-935130-86-4 Paperback

Printed at Lightning Source

FIRST EDITION

www.gratefulsteps.org

To my son, Jonathan

Journey into a ...

Disturbed Mind

Earl Lynn Surrett

Grateful Steps
Asheville, North Carolina

CONTENTS

CHAPTER ONE

—ᴧᴧᴧ—

Traumatic childhood

M Y NAME IS EARL. I STARTED OUT WITH A normal mind. But for most of my life I wished I wasn't born at all.

That start was in Asheville, North Carolina, a much smaller town then than it is now. The second of five—four brothers and one sister—I felt my father showed partiality to each of us in different ways. As for me, I felt he was partial to treating me badly by not listening to me because I was not everything he wanted me to be. As I grew up, I found it hard to get close to him.

I was in second grade when my family moved from Asheville to Union, South Carolina, so my parents could work with my mother's brother and his wife. They opened a bakery. The whole family worked together.

1

I can remember those six months as the best of times, hanging around with ten or more kids all the time. We had a nice home and a great neighborhood. The kids came to my house to play. I liked it.

But like everything else, it came to a bitter end.

***

My aunt and uncle got homesick after a while and decided to move back to Knoxville, Tennessee, where they had been most of their lives. So my family moved there too. I was still in second grade.

But before a year had passed, my parents became unhappy with the big city, and we moved to Powell, Tennessee.

That move marked the beginning of my life in hell.

***

It hurt me and my siblings very badly, leaving our nice home and friends to live in the wreck of a house we moved into. I had decided to put all my emphasis on school to get over the sad feelings.

But another wall came up against me.

Even though I became a straight-A student, the teacher told my mother I daydreamed too much. My momma couldn't figure out how I was making such good grades while staring out the window.

At the end of the third grade, because my dad had a new job as a baker, my family moved back to Asheville to the very same house we had left and had my school records forwarded.

Being back in Asheville triggered a frightening memory. When I had lived in the house the first time, at the age of four, I walked up the front steps and started to open the front door. My older brother chose that exact moment to come out, and the door knocked me off the steps. I fell several feet and landed on top of my head on the concrete block at the bottom of the steps. It took eleven stitches to sew up my head.

That was the beginning of the pain.

***

I now know this as the big turning point in my life, starting a chain of events that eventually led me to use drugs—prescription and illegal—and that in turn, broke down chemicals in my brain and led to the onset of schizophrenia.

Early in the fourth grade, now back in Asheville, my migraine headaches began. My mother consulted several doctors to see what caused them. It seemed to all of them that the blow to my head had caused some sort of brain trauma. Because of the way my brain struck my skull during the fall, they predicted I might develop seizures even though not epileptic. They proposed treatment for three and a half years to solve the problem. I was placed on phenobarbital and Darvocet. On medication, I did not ever have a seizure, but the headaches kept coming. The pain became so severe, I beat my head against things and cried and prayed to God, "Please let me die and be free of the agony in my head."

At that time, with medical technology not what it is today, physicians found no answer but to keep me on the same medication—even though I went in and out of hospitals with persistent symptoms. My family could not afford to send me to a medical center for more advanced studies. My mother couldn't help me any more than she did because she had four other children—a big job—considering my father worked long hours. He drove a State van, transporting blind patients for medical care, and worked for a company making mattresses with box springs.

The next year, my fifth grade teacher and the school principal called my mother in to talk about my daydreaming, headaches and medications. They thought I should be put in a class for slower-learning children and my parents agreed. I felt cheated and betrayed because in the new class, I felt smarter than my classmates, which made me resent the teachers for doing this to me. I felt so ashamed, when each class was over, I waited until the hall cleared before coming out.

At this time I rejected school. I thought my education should be more than just finger painting and playing games. This is when the bottom dropped out from under me.

***

The rest of my years in school, I could not do any of my homework because of the headaches. I got so far behind I couldn't catch up. During this time one doctor did a brain scan on me and told my parents I would eventually outgrow the headaches. I found it hard to believe at the time since they didn't ever seem to improve.

For the three years of junior high, the pain medicine kept me stoned most of the time, especially the first four hours after taking a dose. This brain-out-of-gear problem allowed me to "glide through" since I was in the slow-learning class anyway.

In the tenth grade, when I was fifteen years old, the doctors took me off the medicine. I don't know the reason. Maybe they thought it did not help me. That is when my life went out of control.

When I came off the prescription drugs, I felt so bad, illegal drugs came to the forefront to make up for the loss of the relief I had experienced. In actuality, I had been psychologically addicted to the prescription medicine. In thinking back, I see now that in the mind of a child, seeing that a drug or two can help could start a thought process that other drugs can help. So in my mind, since drugs were drugs, I found substitutes. Pot and LSD helped my headaches and made me feel high, like before, which made me happy again.

But, to my surprise, they made life even worse . . . very rapidly.

At this time, there were not any drugs available to me, so I set out to get them, and, believe me, it was easy to obtain anything I wanted. I soon learned where to find them and who sold them. I was around drugs a lot.

I wanted to see how the different drugs could make me feel. My past seemed so bad I sought ways to run away from it as well as from the pain in my head. A psychiatrist later told me, the amount of drugs I took could in themselves have caused my mental disease to affect me earlier than it might have.

My father worked for the state, driving the blind to and from their work and medical appointments. It didn't bring much income, so he sold night crawlers for extra money, big money. Selling worms provided a second job for him.

We kids helped him find the worms and made enough money to go to buy our clothes for school. I started eleventh grade but dropped out, making money helping pick up crawlers.

***

Then my family life became a disaster. During the time of my illness, my mother and father had problems of their own, unknown to the rest of us in the family. My father started acting crazy. During tantrums, he threw dishes and food. Even while my mother tried to clean this up, he cussed and threw things from the living room to the kitchen, making an even bigger mess.

On Christmas Eve I found a picture of a woman under the floorboard of my dad's truck. My mother had left me in my dad's truck while she went inside the Dollar Store. I showed the picture to my mother when she returned. I wish to this day I hadn't. It turned out to be his girlfriend he had apparently been seeing for several years.

My mother was seeing another man, a very good friend of my father. The two men had the business together of catching the worms and selling them.

When it all began we will never know, but I began noticing this man coming to our home more often when my dad was not at home. My mother cooked for him frequently. What made me begin to wonder was when he came over, he and my mother made me go outside and did not let me back in for periods of time. I knocked, pounded on the door and screamed, "Let me in! Let me in!" Still, they did not.

So one day I told my mom I was going to tell my dad about this. She said, "You better not! Besides, he won't believe you."

Finally, I did tell him. And he did not believe me.

"Stop making things up about your mother," he told me. "She would never do something like that."

He did ask her about it, however.

"It's not true," she had said. "Earl's just mad at me. That's why he said it."

Eventually, he realized I had been telling the truth.

The man who later became my stepdad got very mad at me for telling my dad. He became abusive toward me. "Come walk into the woods with me," he said to me one day. Scared, I went with him. When we got deep into the woods, he slapped me in the face and yelled. "Never get smart with your mother again. And stop telling your dad about me!"

I got away from him and went back to my house. He went to his house next door to us. He was a neighbor. He was a friend of my father. They bought and sold nightcrawlers together. I continued to tell my dad what was going on until finally he came to believe me.

My father threatened to kill my mother several times. This ended one day. Finally she disappeared without a trace to get away from the situation. I was at home sleeping when she left. That morning my dad had gone to work in the company van. She went to the bus station with his car and someone called him to let him know where to find it. Someone, probably my future stepdad, had driven it to the courthouse. We didn't see her again for two years.

After my mother left, the man still came around. He acted like he had no knowledge of her whereabouts, but he apparently continued to visit her at her new location. I later learned she had a place in Tennessee. I had not told my father that Mom had left with our neighbor, because I feared the man.

Then, the next thing we knew, he had disappeared, too. Later, my dad found out they had been together all along. Finally, after my parents divorced, my mother moved back to Asheville and lived with the man. By then my father was dating a woman who became my stepmother.

I love my mother very much. It hurt me very much that in the whole time of her absence, she never tried to see me or even call me on the phone. But she did get in touch with my sister and younger brother. She apparently excluded me out of fear I might tell my daddy. I tried not to hold it against her, but it took me a long time to forgive. I forgave him too, but sometimes my mind wanders back to those sad days. Not only did I have to deal with the headaches that seemed to be slowly driving me crazy, but I also had to cope with losing my family. I had a hard time telling the difference between real and unreal.

I wished the problems of the break-up of my family had been a bad dream so I could awaken to the happy family I once had.

***

My dad was a really good person. He tried to do his best to raise us five children. I realize since he died, he tried to raise us right. In the summertime when school was out, he would take us to his brother and wife's house on Newfound Road near Canton, North Carolina. My two brothers and I and their six children made nine of us all playing together. They had a two-bedroom shack. When it rained, the ceiling leaked. We could look up and see the sky.

I resumed school when my mother left. By this time, my older brother had finished school and moved to Tennessee. This left me and my younger brothers and sister at home alone because my dad stayed gone so much, trying to hunt my mother down. My sister went to stay with aunt. One younger brother (twin of my sister) left to stay with a friend. About six months later father left and moved in with girlfriend four miles away. I was responsible for my next-younger brother. After a couple months, my father moved back in, bringing his girlfriend.

Bad "trips" started before my senior year because of the LSD I was taking. This brought on the first signs of my illness.

CHAPTER TWO

—⁓—

Drugs for Pain

*T*HE DRUGS MASKED MY ILLNESS BUT ALSO aggravated it. I did not recognize the changes. In the neighborhood I encountered bad influences escalating my drug habit. On the one hand, I did not want to take LSD, but on the other hand, I took it because in 1980 everyone was doing it. Given to me at little or no cost, the drug seemed irresistible.

The trips became worse and worse. When I took LSD, I thought people talked about me. This added to the feelings that others made fun of me because of the slow-learner class that had been forced on me for the entire time I attended school. I had been two months short of graduation when I got kicked out because of alcohol use on the high school premises.

This problem reached a significant enough degree to be called "paranoia," I now understand. It became the basic element of my illness. Since LSD worked on the chemicals in my brain, in reality, it put my mind in the same condition as those who have paranoid schizophrenia from other causes.

Paranoia was not the worst of the LSD experiences. The drug affects visual perception—a way of seeing things. For example, I thought the walls were melting and the fiber in the carpet where I sat looked like worms crawling. I thought I saw thousands of them, yet a part of me knew they were not really there. But the part that knows they are not there cannot override the drug effect in the mind, showing these things, so the victim reacts to them from the altered state. Usually when this happened to me, I went into the woods—a particular part of the woods near my house, where my friend Dewayne and I spent our time when high on drugs.

People reading this might see me as just a junkie and believe drugs destroyed my mind. But I am writing this to show something I learned: drugs at an early, critical time, such as during the teens, can cause a significant percentage of those destined to become mentally ill, to become so sooner than anticipated. Since LSD is a hallucinogenic agent, able to mimic the side effects of my underlying, post-traumatic mental condition, too long I remained unaware of what the drug would do to me then and in the future.

I used marijuana but found pot would not totally stop my headaches and sometimes made them worse.

The drugs in the class of "speed" I liked to use most. Back in the late '70s they were given a variety of names, such as "Black Beauties" and "Yellow Jackets." These drugs made me feel electricity went through my hair, and they made me feel I could do anything. I got to a point I took ten pills a day to stay high, and if I did not have them, I became very ill-tempered. To get these drugs I paid a lot of money, so I did odd jobs to fill my need. I even dug graves and covered the departed to feed my habit, a job that later came back to haunt me.

The first sign to me and my father that I had become desperately sick from my illness was my new behavior of running continually. I ran eight miles at a time without stopping. I had so much energy. One of the first signs of paranoid schizophrenia, especially if complicated by bipolar disorder, is a high level of mania. I manifested it as running, mentally and physically. Later, sometimes running away from voices and sometimes chasing them caused me to lose weight—from 165 to 90 pounds—in a very short period of time. At first I thought I had AIDS and would die, but then I realized the cause was just running to and from everything.

The paranoia kept going even after I stopped the illegal drugs. I remember the last day I took acid or any other drug. It was a complete turning point in my life. I went to a different extreme—the Bible took over my life.

***

On a particular day when I was 22 years old, Dewayne and I took a four-way hit of acid, which we had done so many times before. But on this occasion, I began hallucinating more than ever. Dewayne had been my best friend for the preceding four years and had been with me through a lot of situations—good and bad. He had watched me have great trips and some minor bad ones, but on this day, he saw me have the worst trip of my life. He really did not know what to do with me. To me, my mind seemed sucked into hell . . . and for years it stayed there.

I first thought everyone was making fun of me, just like back in that slow-learners class in school. I felt so paranoid I shook and cried uncontrollably. Two girls, both my girlfriends, came driving up to Dewayne and me. The first thing they asked me was, "What's wrong with you, Earl? What's come over you?"

"Go home and straighten up. You need to go home," I responded. But I was the one messed up. They didn't need to do the straightening up.

At that time, not knowing how to help me, Dewayne, pretty high himself, took me to the wooded area where we could get away from society. After thirty minutes, he left me alone to go see his girlfriend, who lived with her momma across the field from where we were.

"Wait!" I called after him. "I'm dying! I'm going to hell." He kept on going. That's what happens in a situation of this magnitude. Others just don't understand how bad it can get.

My illness, combined with the LSD, had me seeing Satan coming to take my soul and spirit into hell for the bad things I had done in my life—doing drugs, skipping school. At the same time, God was on the other side of my head. "I can reach you if you will let Me in," He was telling me. I heard a voice outside my head when no one was around me. It rang through my ears louder than real sounds.

The first voice was that of my father. He said to my ears that were connected to my out-of-control brain, "Earl, son, I told you never to do that acid because it will kill you." I put my hands over my ears to stop his voice but that did no good.

That day with the massive acid dose, I got so scared. *I have to run . . . acid is going to kill me . . . I have to run away from the voices . . . I have to run away from hell.*

I was really running—all through the woods, crossing people's backyards, through creeks and briar patches. I was so paranoid I believed if anyone saw me, they saw Satan and God grappling for my soul. My father's voice kept ringing through my ears as my speed increased.

Finally, as time and space went by, later in the evening, my mind calmed. I promised God if I could come down off that hit, I would quit all drugs. I made it to my house. I grabbed the Bible—for the first time in my life. I read it without ceasing the rest of the night, until I collapsed into sleep in the early hours of the morning.

The next day, I kept reading and reading the Bible, but I could not concentrate. So I went next door to my neighbor whom I had once trusted. He was a Bible man, and

I knew he could protect me from hell. He later became my stepdad.

I stayed there until I felt straightened out. Then I went home and read the Word five to six hours a day, beginning with Genesis and continuing through until I got to Revelation. My favorite part of the Bible was Proverbs because it said it would give me wisdom and I needed wisdom. I knew I was dying and going to the pit to forever be with Satan. At the neighbor's, I could go to the bedroom and lock myself in to be isolated from all demons . . . and humans. For example, on the Fourth of July my neighbors who lived behind my house and up above me on the hillside, started shooting off fireworks in their yard I thought they were shooting at me with guns. I was in my bedroom. I thought they were shooting guns at me. So I hid under my bed, waiting for them to stop and praying not to get hit by a bullet. I took it as a sign that Satan was coming, and he wanted me.

At that time, I was buying drugs. I thought that drug dealers were also after me to kill me. The voices were telling me to join the army or marines to get away from them. So one day I went to the army station to join up. By the time I finished talking to them and telling them why I had to join them, they told me to go see a doctor really fast. But I didn't. I just went back to my dad's house.

At night, God kept talking to me through the voices I heard. The voices said, "All Egyptians are of the devil and all Israelites are of God. I made a decision that my mother, my stepfather, all the people that went to my stepfather's home and myself were Israelites. Israelite people did everything right for God. But my father and his crowd were Egyptian people, who did everything wrong. They cussed, ate meat and basically were low-down people. The meat eating was of the devil, a sign they followed Satan. Even when I was in the hospital later on, I could not eat meat because of the connection it had with Satan. I upchucked every time I tried to eat it.

The Bible was becoming more and more real to me. I took it as it was written. I lay in bed crying because I knew my father and brothers were going to the pits of hell. In contrast, the Bible continued to convince me I was not going to hell because I was a Jew like Jesus.

CHAPTER THREE

———∿∿∿———

Descent into the Unreal

*I*HEARD VOICES REGULARLY NOW. ONE VOICE TOLD me good things about people, but another voice told me bad things about to happen to them. Because of the bad things, I woke up the neighbors, singing in the road in the middle of the night to save these people. About ten or twelve houses had been built on my block. One man got so tired of me he threatened to shoot me if I kept waking him up. That scared me so I went back into my dad's house. But I got a rush when I sang people into heaven—like taking ten hits of speed at the same time.

***

One time I stayed with my brother and his wife. My dad and stepmother had gone on vacation, leaving me at home alone. My brother, Ed, came over after two or three days and asked me to visit him. "Do you want to come stay with me and my wife for a while?"

"Yes." I said. My brother and his family are good people. They tried to help me in any way they could. I really love them a lot, but my illness got me doing bad things to them. It got so I wouldn't talk to them. The chemical imbalance seemed to make me a different person. I guess I really was someone else. *God, I hate this illness.* It seems I was always hurting the ones I loved, doing things that in my right mind I would not even dream of doing. For instance, if a person had hot coffee in his or her hand, I felt I had to have something cold in my hand. It was like two different spirits—an evil spirit and a good spirit—telling me what to do. The good one told me the right thing to do and an evil one told me to do wrong thing.

After I got to his house, he said, "Come play some ball with me and my family, and let's get out somewhere and have some fun. Or is there anything you'd rather do?"

"No!" I screamed. "There are people out there trying to kill me." I could see four men on the railroad tracks visible from Ed's trailer. I knew they were there to kill me.

21

"No one is out there trying to kill you," he said. "Only the family is out there. They want you to come have some fun with them."

"You're lying!" I told him. "I can see them."

He went out to play ball with his family.

I could still see the men. I ran out of the trailer, went through a creek and brier bushes and lost my shoes. When I got to the main highway, I thought everybody in the world was there to kill me. There were no cars at the time. I ran until I came upon a man alongside the road, changing a flat tire on his van.

I looked directly at the man. "They are after me. I need to get home because a bunch of men are out to kill me. Will you take me home to Deaverview Road?" He said he would.

"You have nothing to be afraid of," he said. "I don't see nobody behind you." Even after he told me this, I still looked out the windows to see if I could see the killers running after us as we drove off.

The man took me to my house. My father had returned from vacation. He met us at the door. "Earl thought some men were chasing him," the man said.

When the van driver left, my father asked me what was going on.

"I can't tell you."

"Earl, you can trust me. You can tell your daddy anything."

"I cannot trust you."

"You can."

So I told him about what I thought was going on, and then he started cussing me. "You don't have to worry about those SOBs on top of the hill," he said. "They're not going to kill you! What's wrong with you?"

I never knew why people were out to kill me. The doctors told me later that was part of the chemical imbalance.

***

My brother Ed, whom I had previously stayed with, came over to my house for no apparent reason. I guess I was acting strange because when he approached the house, he asked me, "What is the matter?"

"I'll show you what the matter is," I said. I went to the kitchen, got a butcher knife and went back outside.

"What's wrong?" he asked again.

"I'm going to kill every one of you."

He got scared and left. Would I have tried to kill them, my brother, his wife and their little boy? I don't know. I only know the voices were telling me to kill, kill them all. I do know I have never hurt anyone so far. I can only thank God for this.

I soon left and went to stay with my dad's brother, Uncle Everett.

Weeks later, I came home to my dad's house about one in the morning. I was accompanied by Everett, Jr., my uncle's oldest son. Two of my brothers were there—my youngest brother, Eron, who lived with my dad and his wife, and my older brother, Eric, who had driven in from Knoxville.

Eric noted I had been drinking. "You need to grow up and get a life," he said.

"Yes, get a job, get married," Eron said.

This made me so mad I left. I drove with Everett, Jr., on my Harley to a hamburger place and got me a milkshake. Then I went back to Uncle Everett's house. When I got there, Eric was there, sitting in his truck. My dad was there too, on the porch with my uncle. "Come on over here!" Eric called out. "When are you going to get a life?"

I flew into a rage and threw the milkshake into his face. He jumped out of his truck and started beating me. Finally, I got the best of him, but my dad picked up a broom handle and hit me with it.

"You better not hit him with that stick," my uncle yelled.

My dad quit. But he was not finished with me. I had my motorcycle sitting by a brick wall. After he stopped hitting me, he pushed the bike over the wall. It rolled down a bank. The fall tore it all up.

So I picked up a hammer and set out to beat his Harley. I was going to tear *his* Harley up like he did mine. But he jerked a gun out. "You touch that Harley, and I'll shoot you," he warned.

I stopped and went on into my uncle's house. After my father and brother left, my uncle came in. "Why don't you just move in here with me for a while," he said. "You got a place here with us.

I stayed with him and his wife and my grandmother and his two sons for three or four months. Then I went back home to my father's house.

***

I never knew why people were out to kill me. The doctors told me later that was part of the chemical imbalance.

Here I am, a schizophrenic out of control, and my dad is cussing me about what is going through my head—people that are as real as he is standing there. I was beginning to believe the unreal was real most of the time. Whenever

I went to the grocery store, I went through the woods because I was scared the drug dealers were going to kill me. They weren't.

We had a cat. I thought that cat was supposed to mind me and do as I told it. It didn't, but I thought it did. *Poor kitty.* If I thought it didn't mind me, I picked it up and threw it. I thought I could look at a fly and control it. If I wanted to make it land, it did. It didn't but I thought it did. I went to a house one time and an apple was rotting on the tree. There were bees flying around. I thought I could control the bees with my eyes.

I had to go to court for a DUI. I wasn't staying with Ed then but his wife gave me a ride. That is when I believe things became worse. I went to court but I was losing it. A lady who worked for the state came over and talked to me in the courtroom, "You could have killed someone with that reckless driving," she said. I pled guilty and left. They let me go.

At times when still at my father's house, I sat outside in the middle of the yard and wondered why everyone was going to hell except me. I thought I was living right and they were not. I never forgot these were people I might be able to save. But then, after a while, I had to hide to stop seeing the demons in other people's eyes.

When my friends came to visit, my father told me to run into the bedroom and hide so no one would see me. I would go in my room and shut the door. I used to think he was ashamed of me, but now I believe he was trying to keep me away from their pressure on me to take drugs. I wasn't in the right state of mind to resist.

My stepmother, on the other hand, let me meet people and did not tell me to hide.

***

In the early part of 1985, I knew something was not quite right with me. Living at home with my dad and stepmother, I was hearing voices continuously. In years past, I had a lot of bad headaches. I had them so bad I beat my head against the wall. My mother had taken me to all kinds of doctors and hospitals, but no one knew what was wrong. It was years before I learned that all my headaches could have been connected in some way to what later was diagnosed as schizophrenia.

Because of the way I was coming across, people told me I was having a nervous breakdown, but I thought the head injury I suffered as a kid made me act differently.

Neighbors said, "Go to the hospital, Earl." But I just laughed at them because I knew the way to the cross and they did not.

One day, somebody came to the house, and I thought they were drug dealers who had come to kill me. My next younger brother and his wife are who came in the door. They now lived on Youngs Cove Road off the "mile straight." I had a knife and was stabbing the wall and said I was going to kill them. They left but a couple weeks later I was riding down Youngs Cove Road in my next younger brother's vehicle. He had picked me up to take me to Waffle House. I said, "There's something wrong with me. Do you think it is from when I hit my head as a child?"

"No, John." That is what he called me. "You'll be all right."

"I need to go to the hospital," I said. I knew something was wrong.

"You'll be all right," he said again.

I realized I needed my mother. So when my stepfather came by forty-eight hours later and asked me if I wanted to go to a prayer meeting they were having at their house, I got into the van with my Bible and left with him for Clyde, North Carolina, where he lived with my mother.

While we were driving the sixteen miles from Asheville to his place, he kept asking me what was wrong. I did not say anything. I was not completely out of my mind yet, but after about eight weeks in Clyde at my mother's house, I finally lost it.

CHAPTER FOUR

—~~~—

Life before Treatment

WHEN I WENT TO STAY WITH MY MOTHER AND stepdad in 1985 at age 22, I got "really bad sick." My first cousin, Richard, and sister, Sharon, were staying there too. My mother had a single-wide trailer in which she and Harley, my stepdad, lived. My sister had a camper trailer nearby and my cousin lived in his van.

During the prayer meeting at my mother's house, I lay on my face on the porch in front of everyone and sent the power force out to them and prayed to God for all of us. My stepfather decided to take me to all the big Pentecostal preachers and have them pray for me. My mother accompanied us as did my cousin, who is a Holiness denomination preacher. My mother said, "Richard, you are responsible for Earl. You have to watch him like a hawk."

I wanted to go to church. But I didn't like church.

My family later told me all kinds of things happened to me at these church meetings, which were often tent meetings. I heard voices telling me to lie down. Sometimes they found me lying behind vans or even between people's feet in the middle of the floor. If it were raining outside, my cousin found me lying in mud puddles. One time, my stepdad came out of the tent and got me up. He was rough on me.

What was happening in *my* mind was I had to be forgiven completely to be a part of God. Sometimes in the church or tent revivals, I could not hear myself pray, so I went face-down and prayed any time sin came to my mind. A thousand times a day, I said, "In Jesus name, oh Lord, forgive me. Please forgive me."

When I went to church with my mom and stepdad, it did not help. I attended several churches, believing I was Jesus Christ. I felt convinced that everybody in the world was dead but God; his Son, Jesus Christ; and me. I thought my spirit was on the inside of the dead peoples' bodies. When I was going through this state of mind, I saw the dead rise and Jesus Christ appear in a cloud.

One time, when I went to my mother's church, I walked up the steps and lay down at the top. My stepdad grabbed me by the hair of my head, dragged me down the steps and threw me into his van.

"Stop acting stupid in front of all these people!" he yelled.

I was not acting stupid. I thought life was supposed to be that way. I know now I was having a mental disturbance for which I needed help. He did not seem to care about me, only that I had embarrassed him. I was afraid of him.

He had an old school bus near the trailer, and one day, while everyone was gone, he told me to come there to him. Once inside the bus, he cussed me and pulled a steel bar on me. "Don't get smart with me, Earl," he said gesturing with the bar, "or I'll knock your brains out." I had not said anything to the man.

It got to where I hated being there. My other cousins frequently came to visit, and every time, they sat and made fun of me to my face. They laughed at me. My mom and stepdad did not even try and stop them.

"Take me to my dad," I always asked them.

"We're not going that way," they always said, even when they were.

Richard said things to other family members about me. "Sin is on Earl's mind all the time. He will keep his eyes closed so he can't see sin. One time I took Earl to a donut shop, and he kept his hands over his eyes the whole time. I had to lead him around while he was constantly saying, 'Please, forgive me.' He told me two voices were talking to him at all times—Satan and Jesus—and he had to do extreme measures to get forgiveness from God because of Satan."

Richard was right. I sometimes locked myself up in a back bedroom of my mother's trailer in the middle of summer, in ninety-degree heat, and covered myself with an electric blanket to punish myself so God would cleanse sin out of me. To be level with Jesus, I also had to do the opposite of whatever someone else was doing. An example is: if someone drank something cold, I had to drink something hot. Because Jesus was perfect, I had to be perfect to make others come to God and to eliminate hell.

What I was feeling and seeing I was also reading about in the Bible. For example, my mother and a friend wanted me to get some fresh air and time out of the trailer. So they decided to take me to a creek off the side of a road. I did not get out of the car because I thought I was Daniel from the Old Testament. I was afraid that at the bottom of the hill there were lions that would eat me. One time I thought all people were men. I thought there were men and then there were Woe-men because of what I read in Genesis 2.

Later, my sister, Sharon, told me I had to be watched twenty-four hours a day because they never knew what I might do. One night, when I was in the back room, a voice told me I was John the Baptist. I ran through the trailer and then outside. Richard stayed outside at night to watch out for me and take care of me. I found him lying down in his van and told him who I was. He jumped up and said, "No!" He thought I was my stepdad's big German shepherd. "Go in the house and get some rest," he said when he realized it was me. But I was locked out of the house and went to sleep in a small temporary trailer they made me use. It was cold.

Richard and I often talked all night long about the Bible and God. I wrote sermons and made everyone who came around read them so they would have no excuse when they had to be sent to hell. Baptizing people with the Word was my job, and staying perfect was part of it.

Many times as I was riding in a car, I saw Jesus and Satan walking along through others—as though they were inside of people. I could feel the ray of power coming from their eyes and going straight through me. If it was from Jesus, it made me feel so powerful nothing could stop me. I had the energy of ten men. But if it was from Satan, it threw me into a downward spiral. I shut down from all people and had to get back to my room.

A voice I thought was God quoted to me from 1 John 4, saying: "Greater is he that is in you than he that is in the world." So I was Jesus, and everyone else had to be saved by me.

During this time, I walked out along a highway in front of my mother's trailer. The highway was a busy one with a grassy median strip. That day it was full of traffic.

I watched the people in the cars going by, and I could see death in their faces. I knew they were all going to hell. I thought some of the people were dying even as they drove down the highway. Some were falling dead over their steering wheels, and some cars had no drivers in them at all. So I knew I had to do something.

I grabbed my Bible and ran into the middle of the road to cast out the demons that were in them. My mom and stepdad were screaming for me to get out of the road. Cars on both sides of the highway veered as they tried not to hit me. I tried to stop the traffic. I thought I was God and no cars could hurt me. I believed I had the power to stop the vehicles with my outstretched hand, not knowing it was their brakes doing the job.

Based on witnesses there at the time, cars were sliding off the side of the road, tires were smoking and traffic was backed up on both sides of the highway. They reported a transfer truck came within a few feet of hitting me, but I did not realize it.

I was preaching the Word, and through my eyes, I was sending out beams of salvation to the drivers.

This went on several minutes. I would probably have been killed, but my stepfather came out into the road, slapped me back to reality with his hand across my face three times and dragged me out of danger. He blackened both my eyes and busted my mouth and nose. I was so mad at Harley for slapping me—me being the divine God—I wanted to curse him to hell. But as usual, my mother intervened. She came out of the house with my cousin and I could see she was crying.

"What is wrong with you, Earl?" she asked.

"I am the Most High," I said.

After this incident, I was deathly scared of my stepfather. Every time he walked close to me, I jumped away from him. I was afraid he would beat me again.

***

One day, I saw my mother and sister sitting at the table. Their feet and hands grew hair on them as though they were werewolves. I also saw them shrink and get taller before my eyes.

Soon I thought I was turning into an animal. I could feel and see hair growing all over my skin. I too was turning into a werewolf, it seemed to me. I tried to stop this feeling of losing control of my mind and body, but it was no use. I felt as though someone or something had completely taken over my thoughts. It was scaring me to death.

I could not understand what was happening to me, and my family did not understand. They thought I was going crazy or on drugs. I was not on any drugs at this time of the illusions. Later, the doctors told my father it was a mental condition involving a chemical imbalance.

When I left my werewolf sister and mother and went into the living room, at every window I looked out I saw the devil looking back at us. I thought he was after my mother. "The devil is looking through the windows at you," I told her.

That night, she told me she put anointing oil all around the bedroom window so the devil couldn't get in. "Everything will be all right," she said. "Lie down and go to sleep. You need your rest, son."

***

My mom and stepdad got to where they locked me in my bedroom whenever they left the trailer. All I did was sit there until they came back home. I about starved to death. But when I got out of the room, I wouldn't eat. During this time, I thought I was all kinds of people and could do everything they could do. Once I was Rock Hudson and thought I had AIDS. I even thought I could smell death on my clothes and my body. Then I became Jack Ruby and thought I had killed Oswald. I also was Howard Hughes. As the richest man in the world, I thought I could buy anything I wanted. I really believed I was these people, and no one could tell me otherwise. It was different than if someone were to come to me and tell me, "You are not you but someone else."

"What is the matter with you?" people asked everywhere I went. I said nothing. I put my hands over my ears to stop the voices. They were driving me crazy. I could not think. The voices kept coming to me, sometimes female, sometimes male, telling me what to do or what to say. They controlled my actions and every thought. When I tried to remember things in the past to get my mind off the voices and try to figure out what was going on, I felt like two different people with two different minds, and I could not get straight which person I really was.

At times when I cut the TV on, the people seemed to be talking to me. It scared me so badly I jumped up and cut it off. One time I thought I was an investigator on a dangerous mission for the FBI. Once I was Rod Stewart singing at a televised concert. I could hear the women screaming for me and feel them tearing off my clothes. I saw Peter Jennings "preaching" on TV. He talked about somebody dying, and I thought I had killed the person. I sat there and cried. I also thought I was Billy Graham on my way to the Civic Center to preach to all the people and let them know they were all going to hell if they did not get saved.

It really got bad when I thought I was Jesus Christ and everybody in the world was dead in hell, screaming and crying for me to help them.

At one point, when I was driving down the highway in the rain, I thought I was in Hollywood. Later, when my mind snapped back, I realized I was in Asheville, North

Carolina. Another time, I drove down a road and forgot which side of the road to drive on.

I had dreams of being made out of steel. When I got up to go to the bathroom between naps, I saw myself in the mirror as a muscle man. I strutted around looking at muscles that were not there, and then went back to bed.

The next day, I arose with paranoia about Canton, North Carolina, a town four miles away. I heard a great voice telling me the smell and air of Canton were killing me and the whole world. Canton, a papermill town, lets off a lot of foul-smelling air that goes on for miles. The voice convinced me I needed to go to my dad's house in Asheville, eighteen miles to the east, to make sure he was all right because it was too late for my mother and the others in Canton. I thought they were dying.

I told my stepdad I wanted to go to my dad's home. He took me there, dropping me off at the road where my father lived. I thought all the people whom I loved except my dad and his wife were dead, killed by the Canton pollution—all my school friends, my neighbors, everyone. All the bodies of the dead were buried at their homes, and I could see bugs and flies coming out of the ground where they were lying. I had power over the flying insects—bees, gnats, flies or any other flying thing. I could control them with my eyes. I could make them turn flips or go left or right; they had to follow my eyes wherever I looked. I could not kill them because that was a sin. Even if a black widow spider was lying on me, I let it stay there instead of harming it because there was already enough death around me without me bringing on more of it.

After seeing my father and his wife and assuring myself they were safe, I walked up to the road and rode back to Clyde with my stepdad. Back at my mother's house, I planned to wait out the death sentence coming to everyone. When this decision happened, all the powers I had left me. I was no longer Jesus. I thought death and the grave had won the battle.

This was the beginning of the downward spiral that sent me to the hospital for the first time. Pure paranoia set in as the mania side temporarily left me. I was giving in to the downside of my illness, letting it make me afraid and reacting to things that were not there and not real.

Out of all the things described in this book about the illness, in my opinion, paranoia and depression are the worst once they become chronic. Without the grand illusions and the cycling of the disorder, depression can eat up the sufferer.

I got so sick I did not take care of myself. During this time, family members and friends stopped by to see how I was doing. They knew I was having problems, but they never gave me a ride to the hospital. I stayed in my bedroom all the time.

All the people I saw from the time of the pollution plague in Canton until I was rushed to the hospital were just walking zombies with no spirit in them . . . except for one person at Ingles Grocery Store. My stepfather took me to the store so he could keep an eye on me while he got some food. I was paranoid about all the walking dead who were moving up and down the aisles. But when I got to the check-out counter, the man at the register looked at me with an expression as if he were God. I told him I was Jesus and went running out of the store.

"Why did you run out of the store?" my stepfather asked when we were on our way home.

I did not tell him. I thought he saw what I saw.

This was just three days before my complete crash.

CHAPTER FIVE

—◊—

Help at Last

THE MANIA CAME BACK. I WAS ON THE RUN now and could not keep still. Moving was something I had to keep doing. It was August, the hottest time of the year in Western North Carolina. I was suffering in that trailer from the heat because of my running through the rooms. I would lie on my face and pray to God to let me live. I was two days away from dying, based on what the doctors told my dad after I got to the hospital. They said I was dehydrated and starving and that the stress on my heart was at peak level. My hands and feet drew up and my mouth slobbered.

I had not left the trailer for anything. I had just decided to take the heat and suffer. No one knew what to do with me because I was out of control. The one and only thing that slowed me down was television.

In fact, the night I was taken to the hospital, I had been watching the *I Love Lucy Show*, and it was so intense, I thought I was on the show with the stars. I danced on top of a glass table in front of the TV, and the glass slid all over.

Richard yelled, "Get down from there! If that glass breaks, you're going to be cut all up!"

I did not hear him because I was in that box with those people. I was completely out of my body, and in that show interacting with all the people. But the stars of the show were not the real ones. My mother, stepfather, sister and cousin played the parts. We were doing what the real characters were doing, not what *we* wanted to do or say. I was finally having some fun in this life that I had been sucked up into.

My cousin later said at Memorial Mission Hospital, "Earl was unresponsive to anything in reality. As I kept watching him, he suddenly froze in a stiff, standing position and fell completely back onto the sofa with glazed-over eyes."

People yelled for help because they thought I had suffered a heart attack. What had happened was that while I was on the *I Love Lucy Show*, a commercial came on, advertising a Western movie to follow. I was still in the TV,

43

and when one of the men shot at me, I felt the bullet and fell dead. I went blank for a while, and my mind locked up on me. But then I realized my stepfather was coming in to see what was going on. I stayed dead-like because I remembered the prior time my stepfather had hit me and was afraid he would hit me again.

I learned later my real dad had called and told my stepdad, "If you don't get him some help, I'm going to come out there and kill every one of you."

And so they took me to the hospital.

***

Because of my state—unresponsive, stiff as a board, eyes wide open—they decided to physically pick me up and put me in Richard's van. Since I was shutdown out of fear, they were able to manhandle me and commit me without my consent.

My stepfather grabbed hold of me and carried me to the back of the van where there was a bed to lay me on. While my cousin drove and my mother prayed, my stepfather watched me like a hawk. So I had to stay dead-like. I knew he would beat me if I got up from that bed. But because I knew karate, in my mind I felt prepared for anything about to happen to me.

In reality, I was close to death anyway because of my health, so it was not hard to just lie there. In fact, I drifted away from my enclosure in the van and thought I was in a casket going to the graveyard. I became other people who were already dead. One person I thought I had become was Rock Hudson.

When a paranoid schizophrenic is acting like someone else, it is really happening in his mind. He is thinking, I *am* that person— with all his traits and a bit more. The illness does not let the victim pick and choose what comes to mind. The illness makes the mind act in the way of insanity and the schizophrenic responds to it with whatever things are surrounding him . . . as happened once I reached the hospital.

***

Sometimes I found myself talking out loud to the voices. I would be riding my motorcycle and a voice would say, "Come here to the store" or "Meet me on the mountain" or "Jake is waiting for you at the post office." I would speed up on the bike and chase the voices. I wanted to get to the place and find the speaker. But when I arrived, there was no one there. The voice could be a woman or a man. Sometimes the voice could be several talking at once to each other. I thought they were talking about me. I never recognized a voice as someone I knew.

My stepdad once said, "You'll never be lonely as long as you have the voices talking to you."

"How would you like to take the voices and put them in your head and give me a break for a while?" I had told him.

"Hell, no!" he chuckled. "I'm crazy enough without hearing voices."

We had a good laugh about this, but I thought, *I would never wish this on anyone.* If he could hear these voices for one day, he would not even joke about it. I had heard hell is forever, and I began to think the voices were too.

I hope and pray if there are any parents reading this who have a son or a daughter with signs of this illness, they will not just think it is drugs or a drinking problem but will get them help before it is too late to find out for sure why they are acting this way. It could be an upset in the body's chemistry. A lot of people thought I took drugs or just acted stupid to get attention. So I suffered needlessly for years. If I had medical help sooner, I could have started the right medicine and not suffered so long.

For years I thought I was slowly going crazy and there was no help for me. I lived in hell. I can't completely explain it and can't remember half of it. If now I had to choose between that time and death, I would choose death. At least, when dead there is no pain, I have heard. There was a time I would sit and cry and beg for death to come and take away the battle in my brain between good and bad.

CHAPTER SIX

—⁓—

Schizophrenia

I AM GOING TO DEVOTE SOME TIME AT THIS POINT to the definition of my illness to let people have an idea of what to look for in a family member or close person they know so they can direct them to get professional help. These are some of the things I learned from my doctors, from books and from relatives who suffered with mental disorders.

Schizophrenia is a term for a mental condition involving hearing things, chasing things that aren't there and a variety of other symptoms. Literally, the term means "split mind." But unlike what most people think, schizophrenia does not apply to a split *personality*, in the sense of someone acting like two people. Instead it is a split between reality and the unreal.

Not everybody with the condition gets the same symptoms. Each person is different. Trouble can appear in thoughts, or in the way the schizophrenic sees or hears things differently. The condition can also affect relationships with other people as well as feelings and movement.

When thought is the problem, the illness might be seen might be seen is a failure to make logical connections between words or ideas. That can lead to delusions—believing something that is not true. If the problem is in the way things are seen or heard, the perception of things is what is affected. The condition could appear as hallucinations, particularly hearing voices giving the victim directions. For example, I might have seen a person in front of me who I thought was talking to me, but he or she wasn't *really* talking to me. It would seem like I was reading their thoughts.

If feelings were the problem, emotional reactions to a situation might be inappropriate compared to what other people might do. When my pet rabbit died, I wished he hadn't done that. After I bought him at a pet store, I petted him and fed him until eventually, when I called him he got where he would come to me. But even though I had trained him, I didn't cry when he died. When my Dad died of cancer, on the other hand, I got down on top of him as he lay there on the floor. He was stiff to me. I felt bad. I cried then, more than the other people, even my sisters and brothers.

Some people, when movement disorder is the problem, get a reaction called catatonia where they sit and stare and don't move. I would sit and stare into another world. It would embarrass me, but I couldn't help it. In contrast, some people repeat motions over and over. The only thing I did along that line was run and run and run.

Finally, when relationships are the problem, people with schizophrenia may have difficulties because they are withdrawn. Nowadays I get along with everybody. Even back when I was sick, before treatment, I believe I had good relationships.

Schizophrenia almost always develops before middle age. Typically the first episode takes place during adolescence or young adulthood and tends to be followed by other incidents. Its appearance may be evidenced by a deterioration of work, relationships and personal hygiene.

No simple catalog of symptoms can convey the devastation of the condition. It is the most severe of the major mental illnesses. A schizophrenic's bizarre speech and behavior may cause others to chuckle, but for the victim, they are a product of torment, not playfulness. Commands to act by disembodied voices, isolation by visions of reality unlike that of others and inability to control one's thought make the condition a lonely and frightening experience.

Schizophrenia has no single cause but is probably a combination of factors that vary in degree for each individual.

One contributing factor can be a family tendency. Because identical twins have a higher chance of each having the condition than fraternal twins, a genetic component is suspected, but research has not solved what specifically is being inherited. In my case, my daddy's mother's brother died in a mental institution and my 26-year-old son has been diagnosed with schizophrenia after receiving treatment for thinking the devil is talking to him. I also have a first cousin in a mental institution in Tennessee. He too has been diagnosed with schizophrenia.

Another factor is family environment. Theories include the effects of poverty, maternal ill health and child neglect. In my case, although some aspects of my family life were stressful, such as the multiple moves from state to state, my doctors and I do not see these as significant causes of my schizophrenia.

Although I may have multiple contributing factors, the third category of causes fits my situation best. That is termed "organic." In other words, a physical cause can produce the condition. In my case, one need not look past the severe head trauma, but for other people, it might be disturbed brain chemicals without any known injury.

CHAPTER SEVEN

—⁓—

Multiple Hospitalizations

O VER THE NEXT EIGHT TO NINE YEARS, I WAS
admitted to several area hospitals. It
seemed that each time I was discharged, I
was back in again. The good news is that at
the time of writing this book, I have not been
hospitalized for over twenty years.

**MEMORIAL MISSION HOSPITAL
A FULL-SERVICE REGIONAL HOSPITAL
ASHEVILLE, NORTH CAROLINA, 1985**

When the family took me to Mission
Hospital, they called for the security officers
to take me in. Together with my stepdad the
guards pulled me out of the van, strapped
me to a wheelchair and pushed me into the
Emergency Room.

My mother and stepfather had come in with me but did not stay long. They told the doctors they were going to get my Bible and bring it to me, but they never came back; they just left me there. But at least they gave the staff my dad's phone number.

My dad was not aware I was finally getting help until I was admitted into Memorial Mission Hospital. One of the doctors called my dad. "We have an Earl Surrett up here. Is that your son?"

"Yes, I'll be up there fast as I can."

And he was.

The personnel strapped me into a hospital bed and put me in a room off to itself. As I was lying on the bed, I could see a big monster—a big robot thing coming out of the floor in front of me.

A nurse came in. "What is your name?"

"I'm Rock Hudson." I really thought I was.

My dad came into the room about two hours after I arrived. He was crying. My aunt and uncle had brought him to the hospital. Dad saw my busted nose and two black eyes.

"He went back out to the front and sat down on the steps," my aunt said later. "He told us, 'I'm going to kill that s.o.b. for what he has done to you.'"

He was angry that my stepfather had not helped me but he also harbored a longstanding anger against him for living with my mother.

My father had heard all the things that had been happening to me while I was at my mom and stepdad's home. I had told my dad that day in the Emergency Room about the incident when I went onto the crowded highway, thinking I was God, and how I was beaten by my stepfather.

I wasn't up there overnight—the doctor at Mission determined I needed to go to Broughton in Morganton. It was the nearest state mental hospital

Broughton Hospital
A North Carolina Mental Health Facility
Morganton, North Carolina, 1985

My father wanted to pay the ambulance to take me to the mental hospital, but the law had to take me. I don't know why. I tried kicking the windows out of the police car.

After a time at Broughton, hospital personnel came in and unstrapped me. I lay in the bed like I was still strapped down. They said I could get up. I was afraid to go out in the hallway where a bunch of patients were walking back and forth. I thought the staff would lock me up or strap me back down again. But I got up and let the door open.

That one time I was in the state hospital, I really cannot remember all that took place. It was like I was there in a dream. The voices seemed to have taken over my body as well as my mind. Even after being released, everything stayed a blur. The other times I later went to a hospital I could remember before, during and after. My doctors could not explain a reason for this not being the case with the state hospital. Given how horrible it would be during the other hospital stays, it must have been hell at Broughton for me not to remember it at all.

It seems there were twenty-five or thirty of us walking the hallways, day after day. I was like a zombie. Several days later, I understood where I was—what hospital. When I came to my senses, I was in a waiting room with a TV and stereo.

After three or four days, they told me I was doing better and could go outside and walk around the yard but had to be back at a certain time. Days later, when all were asleep, the male nurses asked me to play cards. Everyone had gone to bed. They invited me to join them in a game of Rook. I played well. They said I'd go home before long. I called my dad, and he came and got me the next day, and I went to live with him. I had finally been judged to be stable after twenty-eight days of medication.

But I was not stable enough to be with my so-called friends who came the same day I returned home. They took me out to celebrate my release and didn't have a second thought about smoking pot and having me smoke it too. After being on the edge so long, pot gave me a mellow feeling of being relaxed and thus the renewed ability to be around people; but this did not come without a price. Instead of seeing the devil in people, I *became* the devil in my mind. I had a hard time. I'm just glad I pulled out of it.

I believed that normal people could see no wrong if I acted badly, but if I turned to God and acted like Him, I felt they thought I was sick. My friends must have been thinking I was pretty damn well the way I was living after Broughton Hospital.

After about three months out of Broughton, I stopped taking my medicine because God came to me in my sleep and told me the medication was killing me. Voices were still part of my life, and I was still listening to them. It took me stopping and starting again four times before I finally realized I always had to take medicine. Without treatment, all

57

the fear and paranoia would come back. I was constantly moving, pacing the floors.

Outpatient Care after Broughton
Blue Ridge Mental Health Center
Asheville, North Carolina: 1985

The Broughton staff had sent me as an outpatient to Blue Ridge Mental Health Clinic. I went there about once a week. The medicine I had been given was not the type I needed to heal my brain initially. It took five more years before doctors found the right one that would bring me under control.

I had a diagnosis of schizophrenia. My illness was also called manic depression by the doctors at Blue Ridge Mental Health Center. The two conditions often coexist. At least, finally, my illness had a name. I had thought I was just going crazy. Was this good to learn the name for my illness and the reason for all my problems?

Even with a name, the voices didn't stop. Once I learned the reason they were there, why couldn't they just leave? This kept running through my mind: *I thought when the doctors discovered the name, the voices would leave because the doctors knew who they are now.* But they never did.

After Broughton, I became worse by the week. I lost all sense of reality and believed God was my doctor, which eventually kept me from going to Blue Ridge Mental Health where my real doctor was. I could have attended for free. It wasn't a money issue but a delusional mind. During that time, I remember going to court with a friend. I saw the judge come into the courtroom, and I felt compelled to tell him, "Judge, you're not my doctor; God is my doctor." He stared at me and proceeded with the case at hand.

During this time of my life, right after dismissal from Broughton, I met my future wife. I was at a supermarket checking out when I noticed a nice-looking girl in front of me. She was buying a six-pack of beer. I told her, "I'll match that six-pack if you'll go out with me."

"Okay," she said. "I'll have to take my baby home and leave her with my mother."

I began an intimate relationship with her two weeks later. We were together twelve years.

Sally had to put up with me because when I met her, I was not taking my medicine; plus, I was drinking much of the time then, too.

For the first two months we were together, I was nice to her. But because of the paranoia, I became jealous and angry for no reason at all. I thought she was running around on me, when in reality, at first, she was not. She loved me enough to stay with me for a while until fear caused her to leave.

***

Just before my second hospital stay, I shouted and preached the end-time message to everyone. I also dug empty graves to be used for people who were not right with God, so they could be taken underground to be sent to hell. The mood swings were as the pendulum swings on a grandfather clock. I would both sing and condemn on the same day, depending on who I was with and what was happening at the time.

At 11 years of age, I had dreamed of being an important person, maybe the president of a big company. But the school had suppressed those thoughts when they put me in the slow classes for daydreaming. They put me with kids I knew I was superior to. My illness caused me to feel in a position of powerful, convincing my mind I was in control.

Back before I married, my wife-to-be was washing clothes at a Laundromat. When I came in to check on her and saw her folding clothes, I thought she was packing to leave me. So I grabbed the basket of clothes and ran down the street with it. I was trying to keep her by taking her clothes. She came up to me in her car and followed me, screaming for me to get in the car. Finally, out of frustration, she hit me with the car to stop me . . . and clothes went flying everywhere. She had to park the car and pick up the clothes while she tried to convince me she was not leaving me, just doing the wash.

Without the proper medicines in my system, my mind would run wide open or in real low gear.

A week later, I had her with me in the car and was driving around. We were going to my dad's house. Somehow, she got so mad at me I told her I was going to run the car off the side of the mountain on Candler Knob Road. I would end our problems and our lives also. She was crying and screaming for me not to do it. For some reason, I decided not to.

When I got to my dad's house, I jerked her out the car window and onto the ground. I had no mercy at that time of my life. My father helped her into the house. I said, "Take me back to the hospital. I ain't right." I didn't go to the hospital then, but I finally did when the law took me.

My dad took me to Blue Ridge. The counselors and doctors wanted to send me to

Neil Dobbins Detoxification & Crisis Center. I didn't go.

The next day, I grabbed a bicycle off someone's porch and rode it down the road. In my mind, I thought I was just borrowing it; but really, I stole it. I rode the bike for several hours straight. I was diving off hills thirty feet high. People were screaming. "Earl, you are going to kill yourself," someone shouted. I paid no attention and kept on going. One time during this bicycle extravaganza, I felt like I was riding a wild horse. But most of the time I just thought I was a professional bike rider.

My dad had to call the police to come and get me because of my strange behavior. When they came to the house, I rode circles around them, all the time telling them how good I was at riding a bicycle.

The police came up with a plan to get me in the car with them. They asked me if I wanted a job at the police station. Once I got into the back seat, they drove me off to jail first but then on to St. Joseph's Hospital to commit me into Copestone, the psychiatric ward.

Copestone First admission
A mental health, in-patient treatment center
St. Joseph's Hospital

Asheville, North Carolina: 1987

My daddy met me at St. Joe's in Asheville where I was admitted to Copestone, a mental ward. The first thing I did when I got to the hospital was ask the nurse to bring me some paper and a pen so I could write Tina Turner and Elvis Presley songs for their new records. This was real to me . . . without a doubt.

The nurse led me into a room that looked like a doctor's office and told me to lie down on the examining table. I did what she said. A few minutes later, a girl came in and told me to take my shirt off. All of a sudden, I became Ted Nugent, the rock star. I thought this girl was trying to seduce me.

"Help!"I yelled and fled from the room. "You cannot have my body!" I shouted back at her as I went running down the hall. I stepped into a patient's room and asked him for help.

"Get a life," the white-haired man retorted.

"I have too many already," I said and took off in the direction of the nurses' station. But finally, a big guy grabbed hold of me. I fought, but he and two or three nurses got the best of me. The man carried me into a secured room and locked the door. I had lost all sense of time and reality at that point.

63

The next morning, four nurses came into the padded room with a bodyguard. They had needles in their hands. The bodyguard held me down, and they shot me up with new medicine. After I had been drugged, I got up and began to cry. They had locked the door when they left. I was trapped. I feared if a fire broke out, I would burn up.

Although the medicine caused me to see the walls roll like waves in an ocean, the fear of burning left me as I got more stoned. I had to lie down on the concrete because the floor came up at me; I thought it was going to squeeze me into the wall. I fell asleep. A whole day went by.

The first thing I saw when I opened my eyes was a nurse peeking through the small window in the door. I slowly got up on my hands and knees and begged this person to let me out. Lost from the world, I was inside a room with the only view, a nurse looking in at me with pity in her eyes. Just a room with four walls and no bed in which to hide my head while people outside were doing as they pleased. Alone in a room with no one or nothing to help me stop the pain in my head, the voices piercing in my brain and telling me my family was gone forever. I was afraid the place would burn down and I was trapped.

It seemed like days before the door flew open and attendants took me into the hall. *Thank you, God, for letting me out.* They led me to a regular room where I stayed for the remainder of my time in the hospital.

After a while, I visited the day room. There I found some paper and pencil. I wrote Tina Turner songs because I knew she was waiting for a new hit. *She needs me to get finished with these songs,* I thought. I found a place under my mattress to hide these great works so no one would know what I was doing. But they got stolen from me.

At first I cussed and raised hell at the nurses for taking my songs, but then I remembered the man in the next room. During the time I had been writing, he was singing songs to God and screaming melodies, and I had thought that was inspiring me to write these hits—the greatest Tina Turner would ever have. I headed for his room to make him pay for stealing my songs, but a nurse stopped me.

"You cannot go in there," she said.

"He has stolen my work," I raved at her, but she threatened to send me back to the padded room with just the four walls. I said I would act right, but for two days I raised hell for my music being gone.

The man who had earlier thrown me into the padded room came and talked to me. "I'm sorry I had to do what I did," he said. "But you were pretty wild at the time."

As I got better, he was the one who took me to the pool room where we shot pool together. He showed me how to work the TV in the day room. People treated me well after this.

At this time, the doctor started me on some new medicine—Pamelor and Klonopin. I noticed no change. I kept asking for Valium, knowing it would make me high. It seemed that no medicine was taking the voices out of my head.

The whole time I was at the hospital, no one had come to see me. My dad was giving my girlfriend a hard time. She was pregnant at the time with my son, Jonathan. He kept insisting she wasn't pregnant; he thought if she were, it would just make a bigger burden for him and the rest of the family. He was ashamed of my condition. He told people who inquired about me that I was off in another state.

Outpatient Care after Copestone
Blue Ridge Mental Health Center
Asheville, North Carolina: 1987

After more than two weeks in St. Joseph's Hospital, the doctor finally released me. He had added one more drug—Haldol. That was a bad decision because I came off it the hard way. I stopped it because I didn't think I needed it; the medication made me weak, and I felt I was going to die. So one day I got fed up and quit taking it. Within two or three days, I went on the run again. A so-called friend came by and brought me some pot and beer. He invited me to get stoned with him. That started a chain reaction leading to a change in my attitude toward life.

I cussed all the time and treated people like trash. For a year and a half, I was the meanest person on earth.

***

I moved in with Sally two weeks after I got out of St. Joseph's. She lived in Kirkwood Apartments. We were together twelve years. We started living together as she carried our baby boy. He was born March 1988.

Sally had to put up with a lot. When I met her, I was not taking my medicine; plus, I was drinking much of the time then, too.

A few weeks after leaving Copestone, I was losing it again. I had obtained a job at a construction site. I was working really hard.

But after a while, my boss said, "Earl, you need to sit down and take a break."

"I'll bring my mattress back in the morning," I told him. "That way I can rest better."

He stared at me. "You really need to take the rest of the day off and go see a doctor."

A couple of fellow workers I had known all my life, and whom I considered my friends, initially rode to work with me. I was the driver. When I stopped at one gas station, I thought I was being given the wrong kind of gas and wouldn't accept it. Of course, I eventually ran out of gas. After a couple days, they would sneak off and take a bus instead of riding home with me.

When I had worked two or three weeks, my boss said he had to let me go until I saw a doctor . . . and then I could come back. I didn't go see a doctor then either. But I finally did when the law took me to one.

***

In 1989 we moved to Riverview Mobile Home, now a family of four with her daughter and our son. Later the same year we moved to Hansel Avenue in another mobile home.

Shortly after the move, my meanness culminated one particular day. I had been drinking and came into the house raving. I jerked the mattress off the bed and took it and the TV outside even though it was raining. It was pouring down.

My wife-to-be tried to stop me and hit me on the hand with an axe handle. When I finally got it away from her, I wrapped it around her chest and nearly broke her ribs. She was laid up for four days. My son was only 12 months old.

All this started because voices were telling me she was running around on me. I was going to put an end to this . . . but what happened instead was that it put me back in Copestone the next day. My maternal aunt, who lived in Asheville, came over and talked me into going to the hospital.

Copestone Second Admission
St. Joseph's Hospital
Asheville, North Carolina: 1989

During my second Copestone admission, I was so depressed I wanted to die and get away from the voices and from life itself. At times my head felt like it was going to blow up. I would put my hands over my ears, trying to stop the voices. I would cry and scream. Dying seemed the only way to stop it all.

Then I got to the point I would sit and cry all the time, even when the voices were not there. I could not understand this. I could not get up and move from one place to another. *What is wrong with me?* I would wonder. *Am I really dying?* This would repeat over and over in my mind, a mind that was needing a break from the voices, but now this was happening to me. *Why?*

Once again, I was at St. Joes, pacing on the fourth floor for the mentally ill. I spent four days and cannot remember a thing that happened. But I know this—the doctors changed my medication again. But they soon had to discontinue one agent because it made my hands draw up. Lithium and Ativan were added at that point.

Care after Copestone Second Admission
Blue Ridge Mental Health Center
Asheville, North Carolina: 1987

As an outpatient, the new medication program worked for a while but it could not hold me down, and I once again came out of control. But this time it happened more slowly.

I began to wonder if there was any medication or anyone out there to help me. My life at this time had become like a mountain highway with a lot of downs and only a few ups with no one to help me stop the ride. I thought that if only people could hear the voices I heard in my head that are not really there or see the images that never seem to fade from my mind . . . then maybe they would understand and maybe they would get me help that worked.

After the second time at Copestone, I was coming around but still wasn't right. My aunt and stepmother helped me keep up with my medicine requirements. I had to go to the doctor at Blue Ridge several times. Sometimes I went because I had appointments and sometimes because I had problems. Over time, I was on about thirty different kinds of medicine. They tried me on everything.

***

I married Sally in 1990 when my son was 2 years old. The ceremony was held outdoors behind Edwin's house. Sally wore a light blue dress. I did not know the minister. He now lived on Deaverview Road. I had moved into a small camp trailer behind my brother's house.

The next year we moved to Lovett Trailer park on the same road.

Pardee Hospital
Psychiatric Unit
Hendersonville, North Carolina: 1991

While living in Lovett Trailer Park, I played music on the radio and TV. The music would talk back to me. I heard voices even more than before. My family did not pay me any attention. I began to develop a bad attitude. I was perfect in my eyes. I was tired of putting up with imperfect people who seemed to be around me most of the time. I thought I was Jesus. Religion came back into my life. I remembered the Bible said a wife is supposed to be under subjugation— which caused me to hit her about every day to keep her straight.

These early times with Sally were mild compared to the situation ahead. As more time passed, it seemed I could treat other people fine, at least most of the time. But with her, I gave her my full wrath when it came over me . . . and at times, I came close to killing her.

I was manic. I worsened to the extent that I could not lie down or sit down. Instead I ran the roads, chasing things that were not there. When I was not running the roads, I rode a motorcycle. I rode it as fast as I could. I am thankful the good Lord was watching over me to keep me from getting killed.

When I lay down at night, I could not sleep. When I got up the next day, voices were telling me to hurt my family. One morning when I woke up, I was freezing.

"Earl, it's eighty degrees outside," my wife insisted. "You shouldn't be cold."

When Sally was in the bathroom, I picked up a hammer that I had hid in the house. I was so hyper. Voices were telling me to do crazy things. Something was pulling . . . pulling . . . pulling me to hurt her. I took the hammer outside and threw it into the woods to keep from killing someone. It has never been found, even by me.

I told myself, *You've got to get help before you do something crazy.*

My wife took me to Blue Ridge. The staff there referred me immediately to Pardee.

After we got out of the car and went in, a secretary greeted us. "Can I help you?"

"Yes, you can," I said. I thought Jesus was in me. "I came to save you from sin and to keep you from going to hell. All of you are my brothers and sisters." Blue Ridge had called and they already knew my name.

"I understand," the woman said.

But she didn't understand. I had lost all thinking.

She sent me upstairs to the inpatient psychiatric ward.

While there, I went outside, sat on a porch and watched airplanes fly by. I was kept at the hospital about two weeks. I kept losing it. Not being able to . . . I can't explain . . . it's scary . . . up one minute, down the next. They were trying to get me in a middle range between the benefits and side effects of the medicine. One day, a female nurse called me into her office. "Earl, do you still hear voices?" she asked.

"No," I lied.

"Do you think about killing your wife with a hammer?"

"No," I answered truthfully.

"I have good news for you. We are going to discharge you from the hospital. Do you have a ride home?"

"Yes."

"Who?"

"I'll get my wife to come get me." I went out into the hallway and called Sally.

"Earl, you're not ready to come home yet. I'm not coming to get you." But she finally came and picked me up.

I was so happy to be discharged. But even though they sent me home on medication, it wasn't the right type yet.

CHAPTER EIGHT

Losses

AFTER THE 1993 BLIZZARD IN WESTERN NORTH Carolina, Sally and I moved to Bradshaw Circle in Candler about six or seven miles away. I had not been in love before, so my thoughts were always in a negative way—mistrust and need to control—although all the while I was really afraid of losing Sally. It kept me being on the offensive. Maybe that's why she looked elsewhere for real love.

I always suspected something whenever I had any idea she might be acting in an other-than-usual way. For example, she might go out on the porch and not come back in when I asked her to. I eventually noticed the same vehicle kept going by: that of a neighbor. I thought he was my friend, but I suspected my wife was having an affair with him.

One day when my wife was cooking supper, I kept waiting and waiting to eat. She said, "Why don't you go up and meet your friend Al?"

I went up to his house, and he picked some greens out of the garden and brought them back to my house with me. She was flirting with him while he was there.

Another time, she said, "Why don't you go to your mother's house?" I left but decided to go back. When I entered the front door, I heard the back door slam. "What's that?" I asked.

"Oh that's nothing," she said. "The door just slammed shut."

A couple days later, her mother came to the house to take her to Wal-Mart. I said, "Why don't you wait till later?"

"Nah, I need to go now," she said. She went out the door as though to go with her mother. "I'll be back in a minute," she called. But I watched out the window and saw her mother leave. I went out the front door and saw Sally was up at Al's house. I went up there. She didn't know I had seen her. I said, "Why don't you come home?"

"I'll be home in a couple hours," she said. "Everything will be okay."

That's when I realized my suspicions had become true. That same year we separated, and she moved in with Al. I begged her to come back. It hurt my feelings, but I didn't give her a hard time. I let her go. I thought, *To heck with it*. The marriage ended in 1996.

***

My dad will always be my hero. He will always be in my heart even though he is dead now—since 2001. He had gallbladder surgery, and about that time learned he had lung cancer that had spread to his brain. He had been having very bad headaches for some time. The doctors told him the headaches were coming from tumors pressing on his brain. He had been getting so any little noise would upset him. He couldn't stand to hear the dog bark, TV voices or even the washing machine running.

At one time after Dad's gallbladder was out, he got really bad. He was in terrible pain. He said he was "hurtin' all over." My brother, Ed, came over from next door and called an ambulance. It was that admission, when the doctors ran several different kinds of tests, that they found out he had lung cancer and it had spread.

My family did not want me to know, fearing how I would react. But one time when I visited my father in the hospital and he seemed very sick, my brother, Eron, broke down while we were in the cafeteria and told me I had a right to know his condition so I could spend more time with him. Eron knew how much I loved my dad. He told me his diagnosis and said the doctors had given him two to six months.

Out of concern for my dad, I didn't say anything to the family there at the hospital. But a week later, at home, when all the family was there, I let them know my real feelings. There were no voices telling me what to say this time. This was me. Me and my anger. I knew what I was saying, and I did not care. "This is a damn shame! Why didn't you tell me? This is my dad. You should have told me! Every time something happens, you tell me about it last."

They all seemed to have the same answer. "We didn't think you should know because of your . . . mental condition." "It's because of your illness."

A part of me understood this, but I still thought I should have been told.

My dad was in and out of the hospital after that. He took radiation treatments frequently. Eventually he became so sick he could hardly speak. It was killing me to see him like this. He had always been there for me, so I was going to be there for him the best I could. I thank God the voices stopped during this time so I could be with him. In fact, I wondered if the voices in my head knew my dad was dying. I kept praying they would stay away so I could be in my right mind if my dad needed me. And for a while, they did . . . only for a while.

My dad seemed to always be in pain. He called out to God to help him and to Jesus not to let him suffer and die like this. He reached the point that he could not watch TV, the only thing that had been left for him to do. He could not even walk, and the only thing he could keep on his stomach was water. But half the time it would not stay down.

Before getting sick, my dad never went to church, but now he read the Bible. It was the last book in his life he picked up. And he prayed every day. I truly believe my dad made his peace with God before he died.

My dad lived two months after he was told he had cancer. One morning at four thirty, he lay down on the floor to see if he could get relief from pain. That is where he died. Finally he was released from his agony. His kidneys had stopped working.

Some of my family came into the room where I was sleeping and told me my dad had died. I hurt so bad! I got up and went into the living room where he was lying on the floor. Because I did not want him to be taken away, I lay across him and could not stop crying. My brothers had to pull me off him so they could carry him to the hearse when it arrived. I really thought I was going to die. I wanted to.

At least during this hard time I was in my right mind, and my last days with dad were a time I can remember. We had spent a lot of time talking, more than ever before, and I was grateful for that.

CHAPTER NINE

Life after Treatment

*A*FTER BEING IN THE HOSPITAL SO MANY times and taking my medicine, I know now what happened. The Bible teaches we should be like Jesus to other people, but in my illness, I took it as reality, so I thought *I* was the real Jesus.

It seemed I always had to be someone famous because of that damn, slow class they put me in—that class I did not deserve. I have been John Kennedy, Ted Nugent, Howard Hughes, Jack Ruby, Lee Harvey Oswald and Elvis; and I wrote Tina Turner's songs. It did not matter to me if people were bad or good, just that they were famous. I only realize this now because of being on medication . . . but not at the time it was happening.

Outpatient Success
Minnie Jones Health Center
A Federally Qualified Health Center of
WNC Community Health Services
1991 – present

As an outpatient, two more years passed before I was put on Clozaril. That straightened me out. I've been doing well on it for twenty-eight years. It has been said to help the sickest of patients. It helps me the most. I am also on lithium and Celexa. These three together are the best treatment I have ever had. I also take a medicine for my tic disorder. There was a time when I would jerk frequently for two or three seconds, sometimes every twenty minutes, sometimes even in my sleep. This has essentially disappeared with treatment. I still have total body jerking symptoms. But only once or twice a day, or even as rarely as once or twice a month.

I also take a cholesterol-lowering medicine and an antihypertensive. So I take five medicines every morning and nine medicines every night. I hate taking them, but every time I don't, I lose it. I have been stable for years. I never had to go back to Broughton since that one time in 1985. I don't think I could handle that again. It about killed me the first time.

I feel like a different man. I know I will never be cured of this illness. But at least it has a name: schizophrenia with bipolar disorder. I thank God for the medications that have helped me. Without them I would still be in a mental hospital or even dead.

Now when I occasionally hear a voice, I got enough sense to know it "ain't right." Somehow the "knowing" seems to keep it away.

Afterword

THE YEAR OF THIS PUBLICATION IS 2014. I AM doing well. The voices slowed down. I learned they were just in my head and I could deal with them. Now I know it is my thinking.

All the people in my extended family were great. Even though they did not understand my illness, I knew if I ever needed them, they would be there.

My siblings have been a help to me, and I love them all. There were many times we did not get along. Some of it was my fault because of my illness. I was a challenge for anyone to get along with. I had my arguments and fights with my brothers and sister. I know at times some felt like killing me, but we always seemed to be able to talk things out . . . most times. I did some crazy things to them, but, although it is hard for me to believe, they still love me.

Acknowledgments

This book would not be possible without the help given to me when I was dangerously ill. I thank my dad and stepmom for looking out for me. My brother and his wife also took care of me, even providing living space. My maternal aunt helped me greatly by driving me to the doctor many times. I am grateful to the medical institutions and their personnel who cared for me, as discussed in this book. I thank Linda North for helping me put my written early drafts and verbal notes in a neater format.

www.ingramcontent.com/pod-product-compliance
Lightning Source LLC
Chambersburg PA
CBHW060513280326
41933CB00014B/2956